T0146656

Poems Promoting
Painless Dying

Poems Promoting Painless Dying

D. B. CLARK

iUniverse

POEMS PROMOTING PAINLESS DYING

iUniverse books may be ordered through booksellers or by contacting:

iUniverse
1663 Liberty Drive
Bloomington, IN 47403
www.iuniverse.com
1-800-Authors (1-800-288-4677)

Because of the dynamic nature of the Internet, any web addresses or links contained in this book may have changed since publication and may no longer be valid. The views expressed in this work are solely those of the author and do not necessarily reflect the views of the publisher, and the publisher hereby disclaims any responsibility for them.

Any people depicted in stock imagery provided by Getty Images are models, and such images are being used for illustrative purposes only. Certain stock imagery © Getty Images.

ISBN: 978-1-5320-9685-3 (sc)
ISBN: 978-1-5320-9686-0 (e)

Print information available on the last page.

iUniverse rev. date: 03/10/2020

Contents

Introduction

I am eighty-six years and still remarkably healthy, meaning my blood-work indicates that I have no illnesses. But that doesn't mean that I have no pain. My pain comes from arthritis and damage to my joints and muscles from excessive athletics as a young man. This book is about my, I believe, clever ways of managing these pains so I will be able to live a long and painless life.

Of course, my desire to master my pain and live a long life suggests that I have reasons to live. I believe that I do. Here are some of those reasons: experiencing various kinds of pleasures. The obvious ones are delicious foods, easy movement, music, art, poetry and, of course, orgasms. But these are all physical. Equally important are the emotional pleasures, such as affection, love, companionship, mutual caring. The most important emotional pleasure is caring for children. If we are normal humans, we would die for our children. And one of the most ethereally pleasurable pleasures is just being with nature, weather it's climbing a mountain trail, walking in the woods, lying in a hammock, or just lying on the grassy ground in your back yard.

So, to summarize, this book describes my attempt to live all the way up to the moment of my death, painlessly. And I will do this in a fun way by using one of my best skills, writing poetry. I hope you enjoy my efforts, and you are inspired to try living painlessly until your own death.

So much for the inspiration, the hard work needed is described in the last poem in this book. It's hard, but I believe it will be worth it.

D. B. Clark

In the poems that you are about to read, I will be my own doctor, describing what I have learned and taught myself about how to achieve painless dying. After I have thoroughly saturated you with this information, I hope I will be able to entertain you with poems about what can make your life worth living before you die painlessly, poems about nature, and about other joyous experiences. I hope this will make reading this book more than just a how-to health book.

Once Again Managing Pain

Again, I'm trying to exist without pain,
Trying to work with the fact
That pain only exits in the brain.
And so, I must manage every act,

So, the pain becomes only a thought,
And not an agony tormenting my flesh,
And thereby I will by my will be taught
That pain is like a babe in a crèche
That need only be lullabied to sleep,
So, it will no longer painfully weep.

*Poems are meant to be read aloud, then you can enjoy them like you enjoy
listening to songs. So, begin reading aloud the following nature poem and
other non-health poems, and I believe you will be glad you did.*

In This Magical Moment, I Walk in the Woods

I walk at dusk through these woods.
Night awaits morning, respecting this magical moment.
Daylight is almost gone,
Softly saying, "Goodbye," before it gently moves on.
But, I am suspended in time,
Knowing that I soon must arrive at the Dawn,
That time cannot be stopped.
And soon I will be gone.
But I have been here, and this cannot be taken from me.
So, once again, I will walk through these woods,
Awaiting the magical dawn.

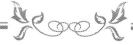

A Little Dirty is better than Too Clean

The human body is composed of forty trillion cells
Inside and on the skin of the body,
And except in cases where faulty genes cause harm,
Most of those cells support good health.

And, what I will tell you next, is no cause for alarm.
On and inside the human body
Are perhaps *more* than forty trillion cells,
And most of these cells also support health,
And those few that don't are managed by the human cells.
It's like culling out the sick cows to ensure a healthy farm.

So, here is what I do to support all these good cells:
Wash my hands in warm soppy water.
Shower in warm water without soap or shampoo.
Ware clean clothes after working.
Rather than using sunscreen, cover with a hat and clothes.
And be careful of under arm deodorant, it might be toxic.

So, long healthy life seekers, be a little unclean.
In other words, in demanding that you be spotless,
Your loving Mommy was being mean.

My Garden of Peace

There is a garden, I know not where,
And the fragrance of flowers is awaiting me there.
And as I hurriedly pass through the welcoming gate,
All rancor and fumes instantly abate.

Then I wander down pathways sheltered by trees,
Feeling refreshed from the heat
By a sweet perfumed breeze,
Until the center of the garden a fountain appears,
Where the water rising there
Fills my glad eyes with tears.

Whereas before, I had never known such peace,
The disharmony beyond the garden
Is commanded to cease.
And I lie by the fountain to sleep without fear,
Awaiting whatever fortune will bring to me here

Pain Undercuts Patience

Pain undercuts patience, *I want relief now!*
Make the misery go away! I don't care how.
Cut it out, cut it off, drug it up, or cast a spell,
Even if you have to make a deal with the one in Hell.

The only thing I'd rather that you did not do,
Is charge me so much money
I'll have none when you are through.
For than my misery would just begin anew.

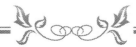

Wind, Moon, Sun, and Rain
A Prayer

Wind, moon, sun and, rain,
The Earth blows round the sun again.
Another year and I'm still here,
Wind, moon, sun and rain.

Milk, meat, fruit, and grain,
Food to feed my knowing brain.
My mind's complete if I can eat
Milk, meat, fruit, and grain.

Wife, child, home, and love,
I only ask of those above,
Where e'er I go I'll always know
Wife, child, home, and love.

Wind, moon, sun, and rain,
My life has passed in love again,
And every year becomes more dear,
Wind, moon, sun, and rain.

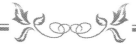

Laughter Makes the Pain Go Away*

Because we didn't evolve to stand upright,
We are doomed to suffer from pain in the back.
But spinal decompression and fusion
Might not reduce the pain,
And we might continually suffer
From a chronic lower back pain attack.

But Doctor David Hanscom insists
That the best treatment is not medical,
But rather, psychological.
And this plan is seen by some of his medical colleges
And almost heretical.

Nevertheless, this is what he suggests musts happen:
The pain sufferer, must first change
From being anxious and then mad
And learn to be rhythmically playful,
Along with others, and finally forgiving.
And then the sufferer will no longer be
So unnecessarily sad.

*Inspired by Dr. David Hanscom's Back in Control: A Spine
Surgeon's Road Map Out of Pain*

Trees Glorious Trees

Strolling through the silent evening woods,
Peace beyond belief envelops me.
Spirits lift when all the painful shoulds
Haunting me let go, and I am free.

Breathing deeply, I fill up with air,
Woodland essence then infuses me,
Now I know *why* I am strolling there—
Underneath these trees I'm *meant to* be.

I am minded of the distant past.
Pagan sires of mine, that hoped to please,
Offered up a sacrifice beneath
Trees they knew were more than trees.

Trees, oh beautiful trees, glorious trees,
What magnificent, living beings these,
Truthfully, I should now use my knees,
Thanking ancient gods for all these trees.

Oak, whose hardy beams are found in ships,
Maple, brilliant red, with sap so sweet,
Endless pancakes pass my eager lips

Poplar blossoms send their fragrant treat
Wafting through the balmy morning air.
Cedar, juniper and fragrant pine
Grace the woods when other trees are bare.

When it's time to worship the Divine,
Fragrant trees are decked with flashing lights.
Children lie beneath those bobbing limbs
Hoping that, beyond those endless nights,
Gifts will satisfy their childish whims.

Cheery, apple, orange and sturdy plum,
Bearing fruit to captivate our eyes,
Somehow, when the early autumn comes,
Mutate into rows of scrumptious pies.

Walnut, redwood, mahogany, and teak,
Gave their all and now live on as chairs,
Beds, and stairs that sometimes creak.
Gifts so rare we pass them to our heirs

Trees that make the greatest sacrifice
Driving out the dark and wintry gloom,
Making then an earthly paradise
Spreading from the hearths of every room.

Oh, you giving trees, you've done so much,
I now praise your life, your passing too,
All my life I've felt your caring touch,
Surely there's nothing you cannot do.

Hear me sing your praise, and when I'm through,
Hear the final gift I'll give to you,
This I'll swear by all the gods is true,
Love of life is what I'll give to you.

Thank you for the rapture you arouse
Trees I love, so when I cease to be,
Scatter round my ashes 'neath your boughs—
I'll give back the love you gave to me.

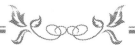

How to Reduce Back Pain without Surgery

A surgeon reduced my back pain
By caging my lower spine.
This somewhat reduced my pain,
But now a more up-to-date spinal surgeon*
Is recommending back pain reduction
Through retraining the brain cells associated with pain,
Rather than through surgery.

He believes that when an attack is imminent,
The brain goes into using the high alert pain cells
That support protective action.
This is normal brain cell activity,
But if surgery seeks to stop that pain,
This session of pain keep the spine
In almost constant pain.
In other words, that spinal surgery was damaging rather than curing me.
This surgeon recommends training the patient
To, morning and evening, recall and then cease thinking
About everything that is upsetting him.
This surgeon states that ample research has demonstrated
That the brain soon has only the normal pain
That is associated with one's age.

I have been doing something similar:
When something is bothering me,
I think about it only as long as
I have thought of all possible solution to what is bothering me.

Then I think about things that I enjoy doing,
Like reading historical novels page after page.
This works for me. I just hadn't thought of myself
As retraining my brain, but I guess that is what I have been doing.
And, yes, I do believe that psychotherapists should train brains
Rather than trying to talk the patient out of hurting.
I guess that makes me less of a psychotherapist and more like a sage.

Dr. David Hanscom

A Walk in the Gentle Rain

What could be more welcoming
Than a walk in a gentle rain,
With droplets that are cool enough
To calm a fevered brain,
But warm enough on my cooling skin
To keep the comfort inside,
On a journey to engage the heart
But too short for a carriage ride.

So I'm glad that I am walking,
And the raindrops are continuing,
And I eagerly turn onto a new twist in the trail
To see what my travels will bring.
But whatever is there, I do not care,
For there's no need to travel this way again,
And whatever troubles might await me there
Will be washed away in the gentle rain.

Pain Undercuts Patience

Pain undercuts patience, *I want relief now!*
Make the misery go away! I don't care how.
Cut it out, cut it off, drug it up, or cast a spell,
Even if you have to make a deal with the one in Hell.

The only thing I'd rather that you did not do,
Is charge me so much money
I'll have none when you are through.
For than my misery would just begin anew.

Leaves could be Snow

The autumn leaves falling from the trees
Looked as though they were falling snow,
But when they fell to the ground,
They couldn't freeze,
So they had nowhere else to go.

Thus they lay slumbering beneath the trees
Until spring enabled them to feed the summer leaves
So that in the fall they could look as though
They again were falling snow.

So Why Not Feel Good?

There is one overriding rule for effective exercising:
Never hurt, and even better, always feel good.
The old rule: No pain, no gain,
Must have been caused by a hole in some trainer's brain.

And when you do something that feels good,
You will want to do it again,
And not just now and then.
And if you discover that continuing
To following the rule also makes you healthier,
And you don't need anyone to tell you
That continuing following this rule you should.

Let There be Winter Again

Let there be winter again.
Spring had sprung like a bouquet of blossoms,
Like a rainbow of color with gold at its end.
And I gathered those beauties,
And swam in their fragrance,
Knowing for certain fortune
Would become mine to spend.

Then summer flowed in with a promise of warmth,
From deep in the earth, a hot thermal spring.

And I bathed in that promise, awaiting its pleasure,
Knowing the joy that pleasure would bring.

But then came the autumn, and leaves began falling,
And the gold began rusting, and changed to despair.
And the beauty of spring,
And the warmth of the summer,
And the pleasure of weather were no longer there.

So let there be winter again.
Though snow will be falling, and wind will be bitter,
And avalanches may be paused
On each treacherous slope,
And I huddle inside, in stark fear of freezing,
In winter, again, there'll be hope.

Meditation Rules

I am sitting cross-legged,
Contemplating my navel
For it appears that Midnight Mounts
Have gotten out of the stable

Now the troops of Lord Anxiety
Are galloping across the plain,
And my stress-strapped body
Is now writhing in pain.

But my navel is awakening
And the chanting of ohm is whispering out,
And I'm on my way to Silent Land
To give Lord Anxiety's troops
An I'll-beat-your-pants off bout.

And now Ohm assures me I will overcome the enemy,
And Nirvana will rule again.
And all that will be left of Lord Anxiety
Will be an old wimp whispering
In some dismal dungeon in my sleeping brain,

Identify the Earth Beneath the Sky

Please oh please identify
With the earth beneath sky,
Be as one with all:
Be the seasons passing by,
Hear the stirring of the morning
As the insects greet the sun,
Feel the stillness of the evening
When the busy day is done,
Sense the roots that stir beneath you
Feeding blossoms in the trees,
Thank the worms that till the soil,
Praise the pollinating bees.
Feel the gentle touch of sunlight
As the dawn turns into day
Climb the trials between the mountains,
Brush the ferns along the way,
Feel the healing summer sunlight,
Winter's chill beneath the moon,
Smell the salty spray uplifting
Near a seaside sandy dune,
Hear the ocean's throaty roaring,
Feel a river flowing by,
Sense the cedar's spicy fragrance
And earth's dark pungent smells,
Taste the tartness from the branches,
Sip the wetness from the wells,
See the verdant valley spreading,
From beneath a lofty ledge,
While below the deer are dancing

Leaping, laughing o're a hedge,
See the forest's rainbow splendor
As the autumn fireworks flair
And the leaves in all their glory
Flutter freely through the air.
Hear the droning katydids,
Watch the fireflies light the night,
Spy the moonlit clouds above you
Drifting slowing out of sight,
Hear a mother bird at nesting
Softly cooing to her mate
As the eggs beneath her body
Warmly wait their hatching-date,
Kneel in wonder at the wholeness
Of the gifts our Earth can give.
Lift your arms in celebration
At the life that you may live
If you do not gouge resources
From the land and from the seas
Making more than should be needed
Of your wasteful luxuries.
Please oh please, I now must beg you
For our children yet to be
So there's something left to leave them,
Something worthy left to see,
Please oh please, by all that's holy,
Hear your soul within you cry,
Please oh please identify—
With the earth beneath the sky

Don't Force, and Heal

Don't try to force the body to heal,
Allow it to heal:
Don't take drugs,
Don't over-stretch,
Don't run long hours.
Instead, meditate, meaning, don't move.
And then take deep breaths,
And then small breaths,
And then no breaths at all.
And after that, if you're extremely patient,
Renewed Health will call.

So, don't try to force the body to heal.
Allow it to heal,
And then have confidence that you will appreciate
What you feel.

Obviously, I must be Patient

What have I learned today?
More ways that I can better manage my pain,
Or the wounds of my careless living
Will make me and invalid again and again.

But more important,
I must now be more wise than impetuous
And willing to wait,
Rather than being always impatient.
My body can only heal itself
If ui an willing to endure
An adequate healing duration

Nature Takes Flight

The sky is red at sunset,
And yellow at dawn.
Blossoms bloom in sunlight,
But are not allowed on the lawn.

But at least the lawn is living,
Although it's so green it seems unreal.
And blossoms that are blooming in the woodlands
Have more spiritual appeal.

Bless you woodland blossoms!
Heaven sends you sunlight,
And after you've rested during the sunlight,
And your blossoms have opened,
Your essences can take their heavenly flight.

Saving the Planet

Since I plan to live a long time, I want my planet to live long too.
Here is my plan for enabling that to happen:

Let the Sun Shine Again!

What happens when the sun doesn't shine?"
Photosynthesis doesn't take Place?
Yes, but more significantly, electric lights do go on,
And fossil fuels take over,
And global warming loses the race.

So, global warming concerned citizens,
Here's what you do:
Turn off all your electrical appliances,
Don't use your car or fly in an airplane.
And go outside and talk to your neighbors,
And encourage them to do the same.
And if they don't yet think you're insane,
Encourage them to vote out
Mitch McConnell so the Senate
Can pass legislation to combat global warming.
But just don't do nothing!
For that wouldn't just be stupid,
It would be tragically alarming!

Plus, by home is covered with solar panels, and as soon as I can affo**rd it,**
I will get an electric car.

Finally!

May my tea be green,
And my chocolate be dark,
And my protein be fish,
And my calories be stark,
And may my exercise be moderate,
And done every day,
And may I never let any worries
Get in my way.

And then I'll be continually healthy
Until my last living day,
At which time, all of my relative,
Who have endured my heath-related bragging,
Will all stand up and happily all shout, "Hooray! Hooray!"

The New Golden Rule

I used to believe in the rule
This too shall pass.
But two unfortunate things tend to happen
While you're waiting for whatever *this* is
To empty out of the glass.

This whatever is possibly going to hurt you,
And therefore you tend not to do it.
Even though you should,
To enable you to hurt not a bit.

And also, whenever you hurt,
Your stress hormones kick in and damage you.
And then you hurt even more.
So, obviously, hurt is not what you should do.

So, may yoy think you should hurt
So you can be a hero and martyr.
But a hero who hurts himself to death,
Won't be a hero very long,
And so a martyr isn't much of a model for the young,
And we can only hope the young are a whole lot smarter.

So here is my new rule to guide you:
Don't hurt, whatever you do!
Then you'll longer and be a good model,
And the young might even want to be like you.

Learn from your Pain

Enduring pain can provide useful information,
But enduring prolonged or unnecessary pain
Might bring honorable elation,
But such pain will also produce self-destructive stress,
And too soon your body will be a damaged mess.

So use your pain wisely,
Them try to live painlessly,
For to do otherwise is not only unwise,
It's is obvious stupidity.

Friendly Fairies would be Fine

I opened the window to see what was outside.
Were there showers, or was there sunshine,
Or was there mostly moonlight
In which friendly fairies sometimes hide?

But then I closed my window and went back to bed
And begin to happily fantasize
About which of these outside realities
Would win my dream-time prize
So I can fall asleep and stay inside
And let whatever might be happening out there,
Reveal itself, or continue to hide.

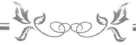

The Exercise Rules

The rule for effective exercise
Is do everything in the middle:
Stretch but don't strain,
Never endure pain,
Exert but never hurt,
Slowly warm up and slowly cool down,
But take very deep breaths,
Except under water, for then you will drown.
Then let out the breath and slowly relax,
And you'll stop terrible tension if it tries its attacks.
And then relax and relax until you are calm,
Until fall fast asleep
And then wake up happy
With no reason to weep.

Till my Last Song has been Sung

Know this of this singer of songs,
Until my last song has been sung,
I will keep singing.
And tell the song-hearers
That the bells will keep ringing
In the ancient cathedril.

And then when my last song is sung,
Let there be a moment of silence,
And then onerestful sigh
As this old singer of songs
Has finally decided to die.

Go at Your Own Pace!

If you want to win the race,
Go at your own pace,
And though you mightn't win,
You won't flop down before you're done.

And one who fails to go at his own pace,
In order to win the race,
Might pay a terrible price,
For doing what he has done.
He'll be lying beyond the finish line,
Feeling like his breathing is crushing his spine.

And though you will not have won,
You'll be the one who has had some fun.

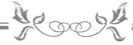

Silence Soothes

It's absolutely still in Shadow Wood forest.
I don't hear birds or bees or even a whispering breeze
Disturbing the silent trees.
And as I've often said before, I love the silence.
So I think I'll fall asleep in my hammock,
And when I eventually go into the house,
I won't even watch television.
I'll shut TV noise, all other sounds in the house
By closing the door.
And then I'll just slip into my bed
And sail off on the sea of dreams
Until I beach myself on an equally silent shore

Health Scientists, Listen to Me

I must run rapidly to catch up with advances in the health sciences,
But the health sciences must also run rapidly
To catch up with what I have learned about
How to effectively go about changing me.
Yes, I am participating in an experiment on only one subject,
But as far as I am concerned, I am the most important subject of all.
And since there are probably other subjects who are much like me,
You health scientists would be wise to heed my clarion call.
So all of you health scientist, listen carefully to me!
You might come to realize that you don't really know everything,
And that your follow up research might prove that what I have learned
About improving my health will be what the new health science *truth* will be.

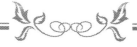

A Happy Life is Not Given,
it is Earned

A mighty eagle was swirling above,
And he called out, "How, old man, have you lived so long?"
And lying on my soft green lawn,
I called back, "Because I eat only the fruit of the earth,
And I drink only the pure spring water that's by the Earth given birth,
And I sleep soundly beside my wife
Until comes the dawn. And so Mighty Eagle,
I have lived so long because Life has been good to me,
And therefore, I wish Life lets it be
That you also live long and happily."

And then the the Great Eagle flew away,
Wondering what he had learned this day.
And what he eventually decided was
This wise old man's happy life was not given to him,
It was earned!

Spring is Good for Walking Too

When the winter snow covers the woods,
Its whiteness hides the brown leaves on the ground,
But is also protects them from the cold,
So that in the spring, their fertilizing powers
For spring flowers will be found.

But now, the snow's whiteness covers all
For those who appreciate the snow's company.
And its whiteness is so overwhelming,
It's like hearing a resounding symphony.

So, let's go wandering in the winter woods
And lean on each as we happily go.
But even if we fall, that will be okay,
For we will make snow angels

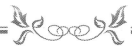

Move or Die

When I wake up in the morning
After a good night's sleep,
If I lie very still, I will feel no pain.
But if I dare to move,
My arthritically racked ancient body
Will feel like it's being belted
By fiery hot rain.

But if I don't move,
I won't be able to drink any water,
And in three days or so
I will end up dead,
And that will turn into a coffin
What had been my painless inducing bed.

So start to move, dummy!
But slowly, and your body will feel
A little or a lot less pain,
And then you will be thankful
That, although you are ancient,
You still have functioning brain.

And then then you should use that brain
To remind yourself
Not to think about tomorrow morning when
You will have to wake up
And go through all of this agony again.

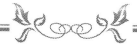

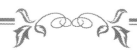

Laughter's the Best Medicine

Let's take a table for two.
You'll take me, and I'll take you.
And I'll have you laughing
Long before we're through.
Then early the next morning,
The surgeon was operating on you,
And after the operation, the surgeon came out
And said he'd done everything that he could do.
And now all that we could do was hope.
But then I told him, that wasn't entirely true.
There was a better treatment
That I knew how to do.
So, I slipped into your room
And began my laughter treatment,
Determined not to cry,
Knowing that if I succeeded in your treatment,
You were not going to die.
And although you were sedated,
I know my message must have carried through,
For inside your marvelous mind
You were loudly laughing,
Just the way you always do.
And so, I told you, let's go out to dinner,
And let us take a table just for two.
And you'll take me, and I'll take you.
And I'll have you laughing
Long before we're through.
And no more surgery will be needed,
No matter what the serous surgeons
Think that they must do.

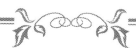

An Active Mind is the Long-living Kind

Why do I keep writing poetry?
Because, like any artist, I must do my work.
Yes, this is true, but now the neuroscientists tell us
That if we don't continue to exercise our brains,
Beyond that inactivity, Alzheimer's is likely to lurk.

So, dummy, keep writing poetry,
While all those non-brain-active old people
Continue not doing what they've been told,
Become even more stupid as they grow old.

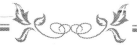

Five or Ninety-Five, have Fun while You're Alive

When I was four plus two,
I asked myself, what's the most fun thing that you want to do?
Well, it depends, I said if I'm old enough
To do anything that when I'm through
That doesn't cause my Mommy
To turn my fanny all black and blue,
I'll know what I want to do.

Now, on the other hand, I'm ninety-five,
And, miraculously, I'm still alive,
And my Mommy is no longer around,
So I can do anything at all.
So, what is the most fun thing I want to do?

Probably, now that I'm a ninety-five year old me,
I can forget about becoming black and blue,
And just do whatever for me is a possibility,
For my Mommy's is in Heaven now, and anything is fun up there,
That is, after one is no longer alive.
So, now that I'm still alive at ninety-five,
And have the possibility of doing whatever I want to do.
So, I'll do that fun thing until my fun-time is through.

Wash your Hands, Silly

After I finished my jelly sandwich,
I climbed up a tree all the way up to its crown.
And then I lost my grip
And fell a very long way down to the ground.

And what did I learn from my climbing?
It's all a matter of timing.
If your hands are coated with jelly,
When you reach the tall tree's crown,
Your fingers will slip,
And you'll lose your grip,
And you'll end hurting your fanny
On anything other than very soft ground.

Shazam! I Am What I Am

I'm moving away from a self-imposed jam
When I move away from what I hope to become
To what I am.

I am no longer the young man who could run very fast,
But I can walk for miles,
And my breathing will still last.

I am relatively healthy for an eighty-three-year-old man.
Although I cannot become immortal
By shouting, "Shazam!"

So, I am not what I was, but it's okay to be just me.
And when I remember to live in the present,
I don't need to live eternally.

But being Too Relaxed could be Boring

There are two natural states of the body.
Tension, which is necessary for effective activity,
And relaxation, which is necessary for recovery
From excessive activity, which is the state
In which most people prefer to be.

The problem is, some people prefer tension.
They want to be so active because being relaxed
Means they aren't making adequate progress,
And they can only be making adequate progress if they are excessively taxed.

So, I guess this means these people will die prematurely,
But that's not for me.
I believe I am wise to have learned to only be somewhat progressive,
And live longer, although of course not eternally.

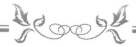

And Mother Nature Serves

When the breeze blows at night,
It lightens the owl's wings
So she can swoop down on careless insects
To bring them back to the chicklets in her nest.
And then it gladden her heart
As each of her chicklets sings.

Thus, all the forest mothers
Rejoice to hear their children sing.
For that the mothers of our Earth
Are lovingly helping their children to grow
Is their most endearing things.

And is it really Necessary?

Anger is both good and bad.
It gives you the strength to fight against a wrong,
But if it goes on too long,
It undermines the immune system.
And if it's too strong,
You can't think you can't think effectively
In order to do to undo the wrong
That has been done to you.

So, manage your anger, and take control.
Don't rage with it, slowly role and climb out of the hole.
That your anger has dug.
And when you have done what was necessary to right the wrong,
Forgive! Holding a grudge, can be just self-destructive as anger,
Particularly if it goes on too long.

I Must Resign Myself to being Eight-three

The formula for my effective resignation
Is reminding myself that, after all, I *am* eighty-three.
And at this age, my body is more fragile than when I was young,
And unpleasant things are likely to happen to me.

So, grin and bear it, old man,
And believe that a blow to your body
Is not a blow, it might be a moment of bliss,
For, next time the inevitable blow might miss.

Walk, Eat An Apple, and Call Me in the Morning

Running, as an exercise,
Might be the popular thing to do,
But moderately vigorous walking
Will also enable you to live your life through.

So, walk every day, and keep the doctor away,
And this will cost somewhat less than all those apples,
And a whole lot less
Than all the doctors you might have to pay.

But I was Really Happy when I was Five

I don't know how or when in injured my wrist.
I only know I woke up in the middle of the night,
And the Pain God was insisting, "You belong to me!"
And I couldn't resist.

And the only excuse I could give myself
Was, Well, old man, you *are* eighty-three,
And an unaware self-injurer
Is what you are doomed to be.
And I will either self-heal
Or the surgeons will take charge again.
To help me become what I could have been.

And, unfortunately, I will have to accept
That this age induced fragility
Is what I have come to be.
So, grow up, old man, you're no longer twenty-five,
But at least be thankful that you *are* still alive.

What Once was Lost

What once was lost has now been found.
And I do not mean that the lost dog
Has been found in a dog pound.
No, I mean my youth that I thought was lost
Has been now been found.

And I know this when I remind myself
That I am now eighty-three
And I can no longer do
What I did when I was twenty-two

Then, I remind myself to do
What I never did when I was young,
Which is thinking and behaving more wisely
And showing compassion when someone is behaving unwisely,
Rather than choosing to despise, which the young too often do.

So, the old saying has been proven true and sound,
What was lost has now been found.

All Aboard, Americans!

I don't love coffee,
But I do love tea,
But drinking alcohol
Would make a monkey out of me.

I shy away from beef,
But I feast upon food from the sea.
And now I'm eating kelp,
And it's making a Brainiac out of me.

So, as far as being healthy is concerned,
I've no reason to complain.
In no time at all,
I'll be developing a new and brilliant brain.

So why am I eating all of this healthy food
Since so many people say that I'm insane?
I guess it's because they think I'm too good to be an American,

Don't be a Fool!

Even when they are intended to do good,
Any foreign substances taken into the body
Are likely to have unfortunate consequences:
Opiates are an obvious example.
And now that marihuana is becoming legalized
For medicinal use for some selected patients,
It is no longer something they shouldn't do,
But something they should.
And a majority of the American public is now
Also accepting marihuana for recreational use,
Whereas it was long thought to be a perilous drug,
An entry into unrecoverable drug addiction—
But compared to tobacco and alcohol,
It is a far lesser abuse!
Nevertheless, it is still a foreign substance,
And just like breathing any form of pollution,
It effects the lungs, and even when taken in a less gaseous form,
It affects the brain.
And research is also finding that driving while on a cannabis high,
Is just like driving while drinking
And since that can kill you, it is equivalent to driving while being insane.
And also, since adolescents who use marihuana
Become less effective in school,
No adolescent should use marihuana
Should always be an unbreakable rule!
So adults, feel free to use marihuana,
But please recognize that there is substantial risk
In experiencing your marihuana bliss,
That you are likely to end up being dead,
Or at the least, being an ignorant fool.

The Old Ways are the Best Ways

The fragrance of flowers fills the air,
And Spring is coming from I know not where.
From Mother Nature, or some more man-made god?
No, from our natural mother, the Goddess of the Fertile Sod.

So, I'll pray on my beads of soon to be sprouting seeds,
And lay down to sleep, without the slightest concern.
For this was how my forefathers taught their children to sleep,
Having faith that Mother Nature would teach them to learn.

Then what will I be?

Why are there not vegetables growing here?
Because they are not needed
Now that my nirvana is near.
My mini-journeys are over,
So, my final journey will be underway.
Then there will be no more desire
During the night nor during the day
When next to nothingness comes into play.

Spring is Good for Walking Too

When the winter snow covers the woods,
Its whiteness hides the brown leaves on the ground,
But is also protects them from the cold,
So that in the spring, their fertilizing powers
For spring flowers will be found.

But now, the snow's whiteness covers all
For those who appreciate the snow's company.
And its whiteness is so overwhelming,
It's like hearing a resounding symphony.

So, let's go wandering in the winter woods
And lean on each as we happily go.
But even if we fall, that will be okay,
For we will make snow angels
In the comforting snow.

Thank You Mother Earth

Being angry with a loved one
Isn't good for him and isn't good for you.
So, if your loved one does something dumb,
Tell him what is a better to do,
And your anger will go away,
And he'll be less likely to do the dumb thing on another day.

If you fear you're going to die,
Pray that there is no Hell,
For, considering the way you've lived,
Hell is where you're fated to dwell.

Monkey see, monkey do,
So, if you're a monkey, this saying is true.
But if you're a man, and this is what you do,
You'd better start doing something new.
If you're inclined to often gamble,
Remember, the house will always win.
And when they see you coming in,
They see that *you* think you're smart,
But they know that you're really dim.

Mother Earth is ever changing herself,
Her ameba, her invertebrates, and her vertebrates,
Such as man, who is the one whom
She has blessed to be able to see these changes.
And what we see what we see today
Is not what we will see tomorrow,
For too many of her creatures will have gone away.

And so we thank you, Mother Earth,
For this gift of continual change.
Now, also grant us the wisdom to continue to be wise
So we will be able to continue living
To witness the Earth through your ever-changing eyes.

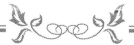

Standing By

I am a healthy eighty-five year old, and I maintain that state
With the assistance of my doctors, my reading medical research,
And the habit of being persistent in my struggle
Until I overcome the medical condition about which I am concerned.
So, when confronted with a new medical condition, I feel confident.
But now I'm faced with another medical situation,
And this is what I've learned:

My wife, Carol, is like me. She is as healthy as she can be,
And she also uses her doctors, but spirituality is her own medical specialty.
Now, she is facing a potential medical difficulty,
But she is confident of achieving a positive eventuality.
Just as I am confident that I will somehow solve my medical problem,
Carol is also confident that she will do the same.
I understand, and respect her confidence, but I do not *feel* her confidence.
So, unfortunately, in this situation, I will never be worry free.

So, what can I do? Ask Carol what she would like me to do,
And do my best to see it through.
Beyond that, this is my problem, and not Carol's.
So, painfully, all I can do is accept the fact that, no matter how hard I try,
I will always just be standing by.

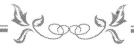

This Too Shall Pass

The wisest of men was asked,
"Why should I continue to live
Now that my loved one has left me,
And I gave all the love I could give?'
And he replied, "This too shall pass."
The wisest of men was asked,
"Why should I endure such pain
When those I've raised destroy themselves,
Over and over again?
And he replied, "This too shall pass."
The wisest of men was asked,
"Why must I cringe and cower
When those I trusted to rule,
Deceive and abuse their power?"
And he replied, "This too shall pass."

So, I will Continue to Breathe

Why do I hold my breath?
Is it so I will not feel what I fear I will feel if I breathe?
And why, on the other hand, do I usually *want* to breathe?
This is so because, without breathing, the simple pleasures of living
Will not be experiences that I will be able to achieve.
So, Old Man Breath-Holder, even experiencing the possibility of pain
Is worthwhile enduring so I can continue to experience the pleasures
Of multiple moments of breath,
Even though continuing to breathe will eventually
Press upon me the possibility of a painful death.

Tea with the Trees, if you Please

Sorry, Darwin, you were only half right,
Living beings don't only compete,
There also cooperate.
And sometimes, as in the case of trees,
They more often mutually participate.

Trees help their fellow trees survive,
Even other species of trees.
And they protect their fellow species trees,
From succumbing to disease.

And they also cooperate with fungi,
Which might attack them,
To protect the totality of their forest.
Otherwise, the future of forests would be grim.

So, Darwin, please reconsider your theory,
Survival of the fittest should now be,
Let us cooperate, you and me,
And join our fellow trees
In having a pleasant cup of tea.

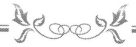

Another Circle of Life

My boat is a blossom that's fallen from a tree
And floated down the short water way until it's reached the sea.
And now I'm bobbing along on inch high waves
Until a murmuring breeze slightly misbehaves,
And dumps tiny me into the welcoming sea.
And am I worried, or even afraid?

No, for I'm a seed, and a hungry sea bird
Will swoop down and make a meal of me.
And then fly me back to the forest
Wherein still lives my mothering tree,
Who will drop another blossom to become the boat
In which another tiny seed will journey to the sea.
And thus another circle of life will come to be.

A Little Dirty is better than Too Clean

The human body is composed of forty trillion cells
Inside and on the skin of the body,
And except in cases where faulty genes cause harm,
Most of those cells support good health.

And, what I will tell you next is no cause for alarm.
On and inside the human body
Are perhaps *more* than forty trillion cells,
And most of these cells also support health,
And those few that don't are managed by the human cells.
It's like culling out the sick cows to ensure a healthy farm.

So, here is what I do to support all these good cells:
Wash my hands in warm soppy water.
Never use disinfectants.
Shower in warm water without soap or shampoo.
Wear clean clothes after working.
Rather than using sunscreen, cover with a hat and clothes.
And be careful of under an arm deodorant, it might be toxic.

So, long healthy life seekers, be a little unclean.
In other words, in demanding that you be spotless,
Your loving Mommy was being lovingly mean.

Shades of Green

The Spring leaves spring forth the brightest of green.
Then the summer leaves become dark
After they leave the Spring leaves still somewhere in between.
And then the Autumn leaves become Technicolor,
Before turning brown and flutter butterfly-like to the ground.
And that leaves the tree branches stripped bare,
And when the wind doesn't stir, there's no sound in the air.

But then, as I hear those stripped branches
As though they are an orchestra's violins being tuned
In a Grand Forest Symphony.
And then the larger branches bang together
As the percussion section,
And from the hollow old branches,
I hear the tuning of the woodwinds,
And now my task as the orchestra's conductor begins.

And so, I take up my baton, and tap twice on the dais
And with a commanding gesture,
I lead the Grand Forest Symphony.
And all the finely tuned forest instruments
Are marvelously following me.
And then the audience of all the forest creatures
Makes the scene,
And what is this symphony we are performing is called?
Shades of Green.

So, I will continue to Breathe

Why do I hold my breath?
Is it so I will not feel what I fear I will feel if I breathe?
And why, on the other hand, do I usually *want* to breathe?
This is so because, without breathing, the simple pleasures of living
Will not be experiences that I will be able to achieve.
So, Old Man Breath-Holder, even experiencing the possibility of pain
Is worthwhile enduring so I can continue to experience the pleasures
Of multiple moments of breath,
Even though continuing to breathe will eventually

My Buddy is a Redwood Tree

I looked down on a tiny two inch sprout
That had grown out of the grown,
And I realized that this tiny plant
Could, one hundred years from now,
Grow into a towering redwood tree.

Just like a tiny embryo had,
Eighty-five year ago, grown into me.
So, I was careful not to step on the sprout
To give it a chance to become what it was meant to be.
Just like fate had not stepped on me.
Likewise, I will certainly not chop down any redwood tree,
For if I tried to, I hope it would fall on me.
That way, this redwood and I will get along comfortably.

Awakening in our Woods

Let's take a walk in our woods
And be entertained by a chorus of crickets and katydids,
And let their music slowly close our eyelids
So the hammock that is waiting for us to arrive
Will sway back and forth, lulling us to sleep.
And then, when the dawn awakens us,
We will be happy to be more than just alive.

Let be what Must be

Let there be lightning,
Followed by thunder.
Let there be hail,
Followed by snow,
The whole land to cover.
Let there be wind
To blow snow away,
Followed by rain
The land again to cover.
Then let the wind
The wetness, blow away.
Then let the sunlight brighten the land
On a mostly dry day.
Then, on the morrow,
Let there be lightning,
Followed by thunder.
And let this continue,
As the Earth continues to spin,
And continues to spin,
And continues to spin.

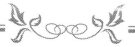

It's Wise not to Hurt

If you hurt as you begin to take your next step,
Don't take that step until you breathe deeply
And then do whatever you can so you don't hurt.

Or if you fear that your next decision
Is going to cause you pain,
Don't take action until you plan a way
To avoid the pain so as to never hurt again.

In behaving these ways,
You will have leaned to be wise,
And, hopefully, you will continue to be wise
For the rest of your days.

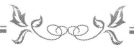

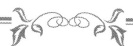

I Must Resign Myself to being Eight-Six

The formula for my effective resignation
Is reminding myself that, after all, I *am* eighty-six,
And at this age, my body is more fragile than when I was young,
And unpleasant things are likely to happen to me.

So, grin and bear it, old man,
And believe that a blow to your body
Is not a blow, it might be a moment of bliss,
For, next time the inevitable blow might miss.

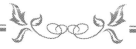

Be Wise, Eagerly Exercise

Yes, exercising is good for you,
It can keep you alive,
But the principle: no pain, no gain is insane,
For if you behave this way,
You will undermine your immune system,
And, prematurely, you will die.

No, the only thing that pain is good for
Is to tell what not to do.
So, stop doing this painful thing
O your life will be prematurely through.

And not only should you not hurt,
You should feel good,
And if you do feel good while exercising,
You will want to continue exercising.

So, be wise, and continue to exercise while feeling good,
For this not a maybe, it's should.

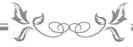

Sing, Mothers, your Childeen are Listening

When the breeze blows at night,
It lightens the owl's wings
To bring them back to the chicklets in her nest.
And then it gladden her heart
As each of her chicklets sings

Thus, all the forest mothers
Rejoice to hear their children sing.
And all the mothers of our Earth
Are lovingly helping their children to grow
And that is their most endearing thing.

If your aging body won't do what it did before,
Don't give up, compensate, compensate.
Do what you can and soon enough,
Your aging body will be able to do even more.

But, eventually, even compensating will have done its best.
And your aging body will be telling you, it's time to rest,
And even compensating
Won't bring you back to effective functioning again,
And accept the fact that you will be joining
Those other no long compensating men.

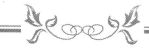

Let There be Winter Again

Let there be winter again.
Spring had sprung like a bouquet of blossoms,
Like a rainbow of color with gold at its end.
And I gathered those beauties,
And swam in their fragrance,
Knowing for certain fortune
Would become mine to spend.

Then summer flowed in with a promise of warmth,
From deep in the earth, a hot thermal spring.
And I bathed in that promise, awaiting its pleasure,
Knowing the joy that pleasure would bring.

But then came the autumn, and leaves began falling,
And the gold began rusting, and changed to despair.
And the beauty of spring,
And the warmth of the summer,
And the pleasure of weather was no longer there.

So let there be winter again.
Though snow will be falling, and wind will be bitter,
And avalanches may be paused
On each treacherous slope,
And I huddle inside, in stark fear of freezing,
In winter, again, there'll be hope.

How to get High without Drugs

Usually you gulp in great gasps of air
When you're exercising and your muscles demand oxygen
But now I've learn I should reverse the process—
Suck in air before my muscles demand oxygen
That's when the air needs to come in.
Then, when I let out the air,
I marvelously relax and feel so good,
I want to exercise again and again.

Painting the Seasons

With hot breath sighing, summer's greenery is dying.
And Autumn's begun bronzing the land.
And the crystalline phantom of Winter waits quietly
To pain over all with its silvering hand.

Though Winters be weary, dark days and dreary,
With nights so much longer than days,
And warmth of the Summer and glory of Autumn,
Seem lost forever in memory's haze.

Yet, I am not sighing, and forget about dying,
Nor am I fearing what Winter will bring.
For I'll paint my memory in blossoming colors
That are spread on the Palette of Spring.

Take That, Oh Death!

Take That, Oh Death!
You thought that only you had marked the course,
Placing overwhelming obstacles along my struggling way,
Knowing I would fall,
Or hoping I wouldn't run at all.

But I ran on, and rose from where I'd fallen—every time.
Oh yes, Oh Death, I heard you jeer and laugh
Though no one ever cheered,
When wan and weary, I struggled home,
A runner smeared with dust and grime.

Yet, Death, I ran the race,
Though always in my own unique and faltering pace,
And in my own-decided time.
And then I broke the tape across my own determined finish line.
So, take that, oh Death—
The important victory is mine!

But this I'll do!

These things I will not do:
Tell a baby how to suckle,
A chef how to cook a stew,
Tell a croupier how to gamble,
A jurist what's not true,
Tell Caruso how to sing,
A robber how to run,
Tell a Gypsy how to bargain,
A punster how to pun,
Tell a widow how to weep,
An old man how to die,
A pastor how to preach,
A Spirit how to fly.
But there is one thing, Doctor,
I, myself, will try,
If you cannot cure me,
I'll tell you how I'll die!

Swinging

Swinging, swinging, and my feet reach up to the sky.
Then suddenly a delightful drop, and the earth is passing by.
Then with a mighty pump, my happy rump
Again is mounting high!
Then I plunge back down, almost touching the ground,
So happy I could cry.

Swinging, swinging, not caring that you think I'm insane.
It feels too good to complain.,
Now singing, singing, I a singing this song while I'm swinging,
Over and over again.

The Healing Garden

When you open the garden gate,
All gloom is left behind.
There's a burst of heart-warming color
That permeates the forlorn mind.

And the air is filled with perfume,
And birds begin to sing,
And the Winter in the outside world
Suddenly turns into spring.

Would that all the of our Earth
Could come in from the pain filled night,
And all wounds we've inflicted upon her
Would be healed by the bright garden light.

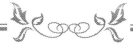

Die Healthy, Doctor Donald

Science and common sense is teaching us
That in order to live longer, more productively, and even pleasurably,
We must exercise, but unfortunately we must realize
That exercise tends to hurt, and if we are not wise,
We tend to be pain-complainers, something that we despise.

So, this is the profound truth that I've just discovered:
I can overcome this dreadful dilemma by creating a process
Of exercising in which I am never in pain,
A process that exercise scientist might think is insane,
But is a process in which there might never be any loss
But a great deal of gain.

So, here is what I do:
I always exercise in a moderately warm place,
While listening to soothing music while in every involved in every form of exercising,
Whether in aerobics or muscle strengthen,
And while exercising, I relax those muscles
By applying portable compression to those muscles
To relax the muscles I am using.
And what do you know, I am not only strengthen those muscles,
There is no muscles abusing.

Sorry, Satan

For all my sins, I'm going to Hell,
And I don't mind it.
After all, I like staying warm,
And Down There, the warmth will never quit.

So, Mister Satan, here I come,
Have all your burning demons standing by.
But don't be too impatient, Mister Satan,
I'm hellishly healthy; it's going to be long time before I die.

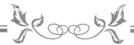

The Wonderfulness of Work

Working is good for your health,
As long you're not working imptiently
And painfully,
For then your health will suffer significantly,
And you will also suffer miserably.

So, *do* work hard all your life,
And if it hasn't been done impatiently
And painfully, then you will also die painlessly.

Granddad's Watching

I used to a run mile and exhausted, sometimes fall down
At the end of the race.
But now I use my old-man walker for no more than ten yards,
But at least I don't end up on the ground.

Of course, I was a young man then,
And I'm an old man now.
So, I guess that means the cycle of life goes round,
And I'm at the end of my cycle, and my grandkids
Are starting a new race.

And considering the quality of their beginnings,
I believe they will have no trouble reaching
What I believe is my exalted place.

So, run grandkids, run, and make me proud.
And perhaps I'll be watching you
From some far away celestial cloud.

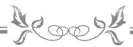

Sing this Song with me

They'll come a time when I must go,
The cells that sustain me will no longer grow,
And you'll gather together to say your goodbyes,
Praying that, although I'm dying,
The best part of me never dies.
And then sadly saying, Farewell, old man,
You have done well.

And then I'll bid all of you Goodbye,
And also, I'll see you in Heaven,
Or maybe in Hell.
But then you'll see that I'm laughing,
For this is my way
Of insisting you that none of you cry.

Then with that final farewell,
I'll be on my way,
And although I'd like hang around,
I just cannot stay.
So, Have a good day,
Fond family, Have a good day.

A Requiem for Pain

Pain should have only one thing to do for you—
To tell you *what not to do.*
And then your interest in pain should be through,
Except if you're a woman in the process of giving birth,
Attempting to *partially* repopulate the human population on Earth,
And in this, no more than two should do for you.

So, pain, pain, stay in your place
After you've told us what not to do.
Then us leave way behind without even a trace.

I Laugh at you, Aging

Don't be the victim of aging,
Be its master.
When your aging body cries out in pain,
Answer it call with laughter.

Then exercise, eat well, adequately rest,
And use your mind to do what it does best:
Understand, explain, and direct your body
To what it must do.
Then your body won't be merely enduring,
It will be blessed.

So, Aging, although you will inevitably win,
And my aging body will never be what it had been,
I will feel no shame.
Instead, I'll shot out, "To Hell with you, Aging!"
As I gloriously go down in flame.

My Good Death

When it time for me to die,
Here's what I want to happen.
I will be in no pain, but I will be totally alert.
My family will gather beside my bed,
And I'll assure them that I do not hurt.
And they should try to control their crying,
Because I have had a full life,
And I have provided for my wife after I've gone
So, I'm ready for my final day,
And then I will peacefully and silently pass away.

There will have been no body-viewing,
And my body is just an object that they will cremate,
After which they will scatter my ashes in the woods surrounding my house.
And then, the will hold an Irish-like wake,
Where they will drink a little whisky and recall all the silly things I had done.
And they will then be able to remember me after I've gone
As a long-lived father who brought into their live, a little bit of sun.

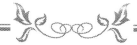

And Tomorrow, He Will Rise

Beat the drums softly,
Donald is coming home.
Prepare his place for resting,
No longer, exhausted, will he roam.

And gather his family about him,
But tell them they are not to weep.
He is willing and happy
To enter his final sleep.

So, say goodnight to Donald,
And close his drowsing eyes,
And know that if it is possible,
Tomorrow, he will rise.

And Then?

And finally, here is this wonderful reality.
In regularly going through the non-painful exercise process,
I am also in pleasure. And so not only do I not mind doing exercise,
I look forward to doing it. And I plan to do these pleasurable exercises
Until my eventually failing body will no longer let me do it.
So, you might even say that the moment when I cease to be
There will have never been a healthier me.

Obviously, this workout requires a lot of equipment that you might not
have, but be creative, create your own workout situation. Whatever it takes,
if you get at least some of what the program offers, it will be worth it.

And a final word to the wise. Does this pain management program
work perfectly? Obviously not. And after all, seeking perfection can
lead to greatness, but it can also lead to pain. So, I continually try the
process, and I regularly fail partially, but I also partially succeed. I
suggest that you try for partial success, and you're likely to succeed.

Other Books by the Author

D. B. Clark is the author of: The Way to Levi, 1stEdition (Kendall Hunt Publishing Co), To Lead the Way, The End of Ohm, The Way Beyond, Self-Development and Transcendence, Ashes to Ashes, A Heaven of Hell, Thoughts Along the Way, The Way Beyond, Mother Rat & Love is Eternal, Left of the Right World, Beyond Forever, On the Shoulder of Giants (all universe, Inc. Forever Young, It could be Verse, Love and Roses, Mercury Smiled, Death: a Second Opinion, Poems from a Smorgasbord Mind, War: A Love-Hate, Relationship, Didactics, Affirmation, My Modern Haiku, Archives Volume One, The Way to L'vei, The Curse of Humorous Verse, These Poems be Philosophy, This Garden Earth,, Chronicle One through Chronicle Thirty-Seven Honoring My Beloved Brother, Modern Metaphysical Verse, Paradise Reconsidered, My Best to You, Once Upon a Time, Wisdom in Verse, Sagacious or Silly Sayings, A Modern Mother Goose, More Medical Mirth, Even More Medical Mirth, Arguing With God, If I Learn, So Can You, A Poetic Fix for Politics, How it Really Happened, Terse Verse is Better Not Worse, Let Us War No More, These are My Best, Modern Aesop fables, Laughing at Myself, Poemmettes, Children Do Play with Dead Things, The New Devil's Dictionary, These are My Latest Best # Three, Four and Five, Once Upon a Time Again, Beyond Forever, Poemettes Three, Who an I, and Why?),The Autobiography of D. B. Clark, Sagacious or Silly Sayings # 2 Expanded, Once Upon a Time Three, These are My Latest Best # Six, My Latest Best # Seven, ((All by Lulu.com)Poems will Make you Wiser, Aging, an Option, Dr Clark's Health Management Plan (These are My Latest Best # Six all, lulu.com),The Autobiography of D. B. Clark, Sagacious or Silly Sayings # 2 Expanded, Once Upon a Time Three, These are My Latest Best # 2, 3, 4, 5, 6, 7,(All by Lulu.com)and Growing Beyond the Fathers (PublishAmerica, Inc).

About the Author

D B. Clark is a retired Clinical Psychologist and college professor who has publish textbooks, novels, and around 90 books of poetry. He has spent 40 years of assisting clients become more effective in living. His attempt to manage his own health is documented in his book, Dr Clark's Health Maintenance Plan.

Also, tread D.B.Clark's dally poems on donald71@allpotry.com where people from all over the would read and praise his poems.

Printed in the United States
By Bookmasters